BREAKING BEHAVIORAL HEALTH BARRIERS IN FAITH-BASED COMMUNITIES

Strategies To Address the Stigma of Mental Health in Churches

ROSE JACKSON-BEAVERS

Prioritybooks Publications

Florissant, Mo 63034

Cover Designed by

Manufactured in the United States of America

Library of Congress Control Number: 2024900145

ISBN – 9780989650205

For information regarding bulk purchase discounts, please get in touch with Prioritybooks Publications at 1-314-306-2972 or beavers_rose@yahoo.com.

CONTENTS

ACKNOWLEDGMENTS

In 2015, I applied for a supervisory position at The Behavioral Health Network of Greater St. Louis, aiding faith-based communities in addressing mental health stigma in Black communities. I was hired to co-create a model for the *Bridges to Care and Recovery Program* they were developing. As the new lead person, I had no idea what God had in store for me. The program was deemed a success, and I ended my career by retiring, speaking to over 4,000 people, and ensuring that 114 churches and hundreds of congregants were trained to help change the stigma on mental health.

I had been training to work in mental health all my life, not as a therapist, but as a consultant to teach people what I knew — that understanding mental health and its impact on our community had to be addressed through the churches. As I continue to train churches, I know it takes a team to ensure that everyone understands the need to address mental health issues.

I am grateful for the tribe that helped me. The people who inspired and assisted me include First Lady Geraldine Smith and the late Carl Smith, Pastor Rosemary Jackson-Moore and Minister Neva Brooks, Dr. Minister Brandy E. Peoples, Dr. Kanika Cunningham, Dr. Pastor Gloristene Morrow, Tamela Wright, Susan Scribner,

Wendy Orson, and Jessica Washington, Dr. Karl Wilson, Pastor Booker T Rice, Dr. Jim Zahnizer, Pastor John Smith, Pastor Jermine Alberty, First Lady Crystal, and Pastor Harmon Swanigan. To my daughter, Adeesha, and husband, Cedric, you have always supported my endeavors both financially and physically. I love you both. To Alexandria Washington, Tamyra Booker, Kendrina and Nikina Booker, Edward Booker, Kendric Collins, Shawon Jackson, Glorina Jackson, Charlotte and Donald White, Regina and Osmund Robinson, Chester and Marian Jackson and Johnaver Booker, you have always been my support system and pushed me to keep going when I thought I couldn't.

Finally, to my mentors, Johnnie Penelton, Mary Rodes, and Mary Stallworth thank you for your encouragement and for spreading the word about my work. Finally, thanks to the churches and pastors who opened their doors and utilized my services to expand or create mental health programs. To my editor, Shelia E. Bell, thank you for making me look good.

I love what I do. This book is a compilation of what I've learned and found effective in my daily endeavors for eight years as the director of faith-based initiatives for the Behavioral Health Network. I've utilized this information in training churches nationwide.

As a result, I created a new component for my work. In January 2023, my latest program to continue the ministry I love provides training and technical assistance to churches nationwide. As of June 2023, I began providing further consultation through the Breaking Behavioral-Health Barriers (BBB) Faith Project. The program emphasizes the importance of congregations participating in behavioral health training to ensure churches understand how to support people in an emergency and are ready to respond and assist before they are in crisis. Finally, I was recently certified as a professional Christian mental health coach and have enrolled in seminary school to pursue my doctorate in ministry. I will receive my Doctorate in Practical Ministry and Counseling in January 2024.

I dedicate this book to my only grandson,

ISAIAH

FOREWORD

Several years ago, I had the pleasure of meeting Rose Jackson-Beavers. Back then, our initial conversation at a local coffee shop seemed like just that – a casual chat. Little did I know that it would evolve into a mentorship, partnership, and, most importantly, a deep and enduring friendship.

In the time since, I've come to recognize Ms. Rose, as I affectionately call her, as the ultimate authority when it comes to understanding mental health, especially within faith-based organizations. She's the "go-to" person, and our collaboration on various projects has only solidified this truth. Ms. Rose's passion and purpose precede her, making her a well-known figure in the community.

For years, she has dedicated herself to building relationships with hundreds of churches, diligently training pastors and parishioners on the critical importance of creating behavioral health-friendly environments. As I mentioned before, she is the one people turn to. Ms. Rose not only possesses the education and experience required for this work but, crucially, she genuinely cares about ensuring individuals get the help they deeply need.

Moreover, Ms. Rose's influence extends beyond the projects we've undertaken together. Her commitment to destigmatizing mental health in the black community is a beacon of inspiration. I've witnessed her tireless efforts to challenge preconceptions and encourage open dialogue within churches, creating spaces where individuals feel seen, heard, and understood. This book not only reflects Ms. Rose's profound impact but also stands as a call to action. May it ignite conversations, prompt self-reflection, and empower communities to embrace the transformative power of mental health awareness.

Rose's book, 'Breaking Behavioral Health Barriers in Faith-based Communities' is a testament to Ms. Rose's dedication. I hope it serves as a valuable tool for others on their collective and individual journeys toward what she values most – mental, emotional, and spiritual wholeness.

Dr. Brandy S. Peoples
Psychologist

"And we know that all things work together for good to them that love God, to them who are the called according to his purpose."

ROMANS 8:28

THE BEGINNING OF MY ROAD TO
MENTAL HEALTH TRAINING

In the early stages of my career, I held the position of Mental Health Coordinator. My primary responsibility was to address employee burnout within the organization. To achieve this, I arranged for therapists to engage with our staff and the families we served regularly. Planning events involved inviting therapists to conduct workshops and mental health and well-being activities. Additionally, I organized team-building events such as skating outings and dinners, all approved by the company. The aim was simple: if we could keep our staff and the families we served content and mentally healthy, we would have a higher employee retention rate. I cherished this role, even though it was relatively short-lived. After one year, I was promoted to Case Management Coordinator. However, my journey to support mental health persisted, eventually leading me to work with churches.

My lifelong commitment to enhancing mental health and overall well-being started in my home. My mother instilled in us the importance of caring for physical and mental health. I vividly recall having conversations with her about mental health matters from a very young age. My mother emphasized that seeking counseling from a licensed professional was not a sign of weakness but a path to healing and growth. She pointed to characters on television shows like "The Young and the Restless," where characters openly discussed therapy and its positive impact. While the characters may not have explicitly addressed mental health, they conveyed that therapy was beneficial. This simple observation sparked a crucial realization that therapy could be a source of healing. Mom's perspective was that even the wealthy considered therapy a badge of honor. From this, I learned that discussing mental health was necessary and expected. My mother's encouragement was not limited to mental health but extended to our spiritual lives as well. Just as prayer was essential, counseling was equally valuable.

Between the ages of 10 and 12, my mother took her daughters to meet her therapist. During that visit, I was captivated by the power and significance of the psychiatrist who sat before us, asking questions with the intention of understanding and healing. The doctor's purpose for meeting us was simple: to meet the children who brought joy and fulfillment to her patient's life. It was a pivotal moment, and I left the session with a beaming smile. I knew then that I wanted to make a difference in the field of mental health, just as that psychiatrist did.

As the years went by, I found myself following in my mother's footsteps, helping those around me. My first experience involved mediating an argument between my parents and offering an early intervention to prevent further conflict. Recognizing the positive impact of counseling, I contacted my uncle, Herod, to provide spiritual guidance when my parents' arguments escalated. It was clear that talking about problems and seeking help, whether spiritual or therapeutic, could make a significant difference in people's lives.

Over the years, I have been consulted by people from across the country eager to establish behavioral health ministries in their churches. This endeavor was incredibly close to my heart because churches historically emphasized physical health and prayer, often overlooking the topic of mental health. A significant disconnect existed between the Christian faith and mental health, with many people erroneously believing that seeking counseling implied a lack of faith in God.

My conviction was that God grants us various talents and expects us to use them to help others. Thus, I delved into understanding the origins of the stigma surrounding mental health in the Christian context. God desires us to be whole in spirit, body, and soul, so why weren't we teaching people to care for their entire well-being, including mental health?

For instance, I once encountered an intelligent man with a high-ranking position in the St. Louis and Illinois metropolitan communities. When I suggested that children needed resources like counseling to address the trauma they were experiencing, he dismissed the idea. He firmly believed that children needed only to pray, viewing social workers' suggestions for counseling as unnecessary. The truth is that people in trauma require both counseling *and* prayer, as this combination can fortify their resolve to recover and assure them that God is working on their behalf.

Years later, I found the words to convey my perspective to other church members with similar beliefs. When faced with such beliefs, I share the Bible verse 1 Thessalonians 5:23, which underscores God's desire for our holistic well-being, including spiritual, physical, and mental health. I present that if God wants us to be whole, the church must help its members achieve that wholeness.

This book sheds light on my journey to becoming a professional trainer in the faith-based community. I hope it encourages churches to promote comprehensive well-being, encompassing spiritual and mental health, and not just prayer alone.

"For God hath not given us the spirit of fear; but of power, and of love, and of a sound mind."

2 TIMOTHY 1:7

ONE

Changing Our View on Mental Health

There exists a pervasive historical bias surrounding mental health, perpetuating misconceptions and fostering fear. Unfortunately, many individuals lack a comprehensive understanding of what mental health entails, often reducing it to a stereotype of "craziness." Fear of the unknown tends to exacerbate this lack of knowledge, hindering the development of a nuanced perspective.

Mental health encompasses conditions affecting a person's thinking, feeling, or mood, influencing their ability to relate to others and function daily. It is crucial to recognize the diversity of experiences within the realm of mental health to dispel intimidation and promote acceptance of treatment. With over 200 classified forms of mental illness, common disorders include bipolar disorder, clinical depression, dementia, schizophrenia, and anxiety disorders. While some may associate certain conditions with being "messed up in the head," it is imperative to acknowledge the varied nature of these disorders. Labeling individuals as "crazy" only obstructs their path to seeking help.

Understanding the multitude of mental disorders is vital, yet societal indifference persists, perpetuated by the invisibility of those suffering. Cultural norms, family traditions, and societal expectations contribute to the silence surrounding mental health discussions. Understanding different disorders and their symptoms is essential to bridge this gap. Spending time around individuals with mental health challenges reveals observable changes in behavior, including mood swings, personality shifts, altered personal habits, and social withdrawal.

As a former director of a faith-based initiative, I encountered numerous calls on our hotline, predominantly related to common mental health disorders such as grief, anxiety, depression, and bipolar disorder. Recognizing these patterns enables us to appreciate the importance of education and awareness in addressing behavioral health issues.

Why, then, do so many individuals miss the mark in comprehending the significance of mental health understanding? Examining biblical narratives reveals numerous instances of trauma, offering parallels to the challenges faced by those with mental health disorders. However, historical myths, societal biases, and familial stigmas perpetuate the reluctance to seek mental health support.

The stigma surrounding mental illness is universal, yet when personally affected, individuals often feel isolated. Addressing mental health in communities necessitates confronting the pervasive stigma that manifests as harmful and unfair beliefs, creating a mark of shame or discredit.

Reflecting on a personal childhood experience underscores the impact of stigma. A young boy, seemingly mentally challenged, faced derogatory comments and name-calling from peers. This incident, shaped by ignorance, highlights the need for empathy, understanding, and the harmful consequences of perpetuating societal biases.

Community phrases like "whatever happens in the home, stays in the home" further contribute to the veil of silence surrounding mental health. Individuals with undiagnosed mental illnesses often remain hidden away, a practice reinforced by familial expectations. The secrecy and fear surrounding mental health conditions can create a barrier to understanding and compassion.

Education and awareness are pivotal in dismantling the historical misperceptions of mental health. The portrayal of special education classrooms and segregated school buses for those with mental health challenges perpetuates stereotypes, fostering an environment of mistreatment and alienation. Mental illness should be viewed like any other disease, devoid of the unfounded fear that one can *catch it* merely by association.

Recognizing the diversity of mental health experiences, dispelling stereotypes, and promoting education are crucial steps in fostering a healthier, more compassionate society. By challenging historical biases and encouraging open conversations, we can break the silence surrounding mental health and create a supportive environment for individuals and families affected by mental health challenges.

"Where no counsel is, the people fall: but in the multitude of counsellors there is safety."

PROVERBS 11:14

TWO

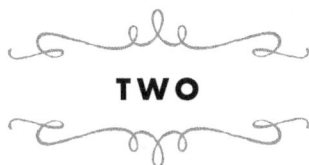

Ensuring Churches Have Vital Information, Awareness, and Resources

In the pursuit of sound healthcare decisions, it becomes essential to cultivate a reservoir of knowledge. It is imperative to actively research and seek resources to enhance our understanding of the intricacies of mental and physical health. Often, we need to pay more attention to the importance of comprehending the inner workings of our minds and bodies. When our homes, schools, or churches fail to provide education, we are adrift in a sea of ignorance. Failing to grasp the implications of our ignorance can be detrimental to our well-being, especially when specific communities face unique barriers to accessing healthcare.

Education plays a pivotal role in illuminating the path toward a brighter future. It is the cornerstone for change, especially in communities where the stigma around mental health looms large. By instilling knowledge of the value of mental health, the various treatment options, and the possibility of recovery, more individuals may be encouraged to seek help without fear of repercussions. Yet, our challenge lies in fostering these essential conversations in our homes and communities.

By providing education, we can dispel negative stereotypes and connotations associated with mental health. This transformation starts at the heart of our communities—our churches. Churches have a unique opportunity to host mental health education for their congregants. Such efforts go beyond mere service; they represent a form of pastoral care that signals acceptance and support. While many churches prioritize physical health, the significance of mental health should not be understated. The brain, often called the seat of intelligence, is crucial in guiding our emotions, sensations, movements, and behavior. It is one of the main vital organs in our bodies, and understanding its importance should drive the planning of church activities. However, I observed that mental health programming in churches remains scarce. Physical activities are common, but mental health services are largely absent.

In the journey to better health, churches should couple their focus on physical well-being with an equal commitment to mental health support. This two-pronged approach aligns with the core teachings of love and care. It is essential to equip congregants with the tools they need for a holistic approach to health. In this context, "tools" encompass many resources, practices, and activities that promote physical, mental, and spiritual well-being. From information to self-care activities, exercise, scriptures, and training, these tools enhance the ability to manage stress, find contentment, and achieve overall well-being. They serve as a means to empower individuals with the knowledge and understanding required to confront the complexities of mental health.

Awareness, the second building block, ensures people are mindful of mental health matters. To be aware requires a concerted effort by churches to educate their members through seminars, social events, and networking with mental health-focused agencies. Engaging in activities such as hosting health fairs, distributing brochures, and inviting guest speakers can provide valuable insights. Even pastors can play a vital role by addressing mental health from the pulpit, drawing on stories from the Bible that tackle trauma. The goal is to ensure that the church and the community remain informed about mental health, self-care, and grief management. This effort necessitates a multipronged approach, with numerous ways to keep church members and the community aware of these critical topics.

Equipping churches with the tools for behavioral health training is essential to prepare them to address mental health effectively. These physical and informational tools are long-lasting resources that, when used consistently, are helpful. The adage "teach a man to fish, and he can eat for a lifetime" rings true in the context of mental health. New members should be given access to these tools to help them navigate available resources and stay informed about current mental health issues. These tools encompass everything from self-care activities to information dissemination and mental health training. They empower congregants to care for themselves and enhance their church's well-being, strengthening faith and mental health bonds.

Ultimately, churches play a pivotal role in reducing the stigma surrounding mental health and preparing individuals to address these issues within their families and personally. As important community access points, churches should be ready to address all social concerns and issues affecting their congregants, their families, and the community. When people possess the essential triad of information, awareness, and tools to comprehend prevalent issues in their homes and communities, they become better equipped to address these concerns without fear. This transformation is critical to reducing stigma and encouraging individuals to seek help when needed. With these tools and understanding, individuals can take control of their emotions and actions, knowing that resources are available to alleviate their pain, fears, and lack of understanding.

"And the very God of peace sanctify you wholly; and I pray God your whole spirit and soul and body be preserved blameless unto the coming of our Lord Jesus Christ."

1 THESSALONIANS 5:23

THREE

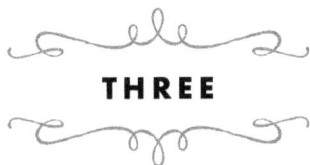

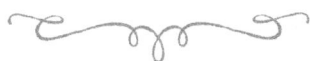

Embracing God's Vision of Wholeness

Mental illness is a significant part of this broken world. It encompasses conditions affecting an individual's thinking, feeling, or mood, potentially impacting their ability to relate to others and function daily.

From a young age, the importance of health was instilled in me by our church and my mother. As a devoted Adventist, our faith community emphasized the significance of healthy living. We adhered to the guidance in 1 Corinthians 10:31: "So, whether you eat or drink, or whatever you do, do all to the glory of God." While interpretations may vary, for my family, this meant safeguarding God's temple. It meant making conscious choices in eating and drinking and recognizing that detrimental habits could negatively impact our well-being. Matthew 6:34 reinforced this perspective: "So do not worry about tomorrow; for tomorrow will care for itself. Each day has enough trouble of its own." We were encouraged to cast our anxieties upon God, trusting He cared for us and would provide.

In the Book of Genesis, we learn that God created humanity in a state of holistic health, where physical, emotional, and spiritual well-being were united. The fall of Adam and Eve marked a departure from this wholeness, introducing dysfunction and diseases into our world.

The Bible doesn't mention "mental health," yet its narratives are replete with instances of people grappling with inner turmoil. They endured experiences that stirred feelings of depression, anxiety, and more. Deuteronomy 28:28 carries a stark warning from God: "The Lord will strike you with madness and blindness and confusion of heart." This passage emphasizes the potential consequences of disobedience and hints at a link between disobedience and mental health struggles.

The Bible is rich with accounts of individuals who exhibited symptoms of anxiety and depression. For example, consider Jonah's experience within the belly of a fish, enduring uncertainty and isolation due to his disobedience. The Book of Ruth depicts Naomi's sorrow after losing her husband and two sons. These stories provide glimpses into the human experiences of trauma and depression, even in biblical times.

Many individuals grapple with mental health issues, yet stigma often compels them to conceal their struggles behind closed doors. It is vital to confront this issue openly and remind people that it is not their fault. They are not broken, and with treatment, recovery is possible.

Society's attitudes and misconceptions around mental health often drive individuals to hide their pain. Fear of judgment and a lack of knowledge prevent them from seeking help. As a result, many issues go unaddressed. Statistics reveal the prevalence of mental health struggles, with approximately 1 in 5 U.S. adults experiencing mental illness each year. An estimated 50% of all lifetime mental illness begins by age 14, emphasizing the need to acknowledge and support those facing mental health challenges.[1] It is imperative to understand that love transcends boundaries, and by helping others during their difficult times, we sow seeds of kindness and support.

The church plays a vital role in the lives of many African Americans, from spiritual guidance to community support and education. As a haven and a source of stability, the church must be ready to offer resources and referrals for mental health. The journey toward wholeness requires the church to establish a behavioral health-friendly ministry.

1 Thessalonians 5:23, we are called to promote wholeness in spirit, soul, and body. God expects that we share information with those in distress, ensuring they receive the help they need. Just as we take care of our physical bodies, tending to ailments and discomfort, we must be equally attentive to the state of our minds. Our faith tradition emphasizes the importance of caring for the whole being, echoing verses that refer to our bodies as temples. God's concern encompasses our spiritual, mental, and physical well-being. This perspective encourages us to become peacemakers, extending

---

[1] https://www.nimb.nih.gov/health/statistics/mentalillness

kindness and aid to those in need, especially the marginalized and oppressed.

Pastors must understand that stigma prevents many individuals from disclosing their struggles, and it is essential to be prepared to support those who reach out for comfort and information. As we await the day we'll be made whole in God's presence, we must tend to our physical, mental, and spiritual well-being. This means caring for our bodies, nourishing our minds, and practicing self-care. When we're unwell, seeking medical and mental health care is appropriate. Proverbs 19:20 wisely reminds us, "Hear counsel, and receive instruction, that thou mayest be wise in thy latter end."

Here are a few passages that are often discussed about mental health:

1 Thessalonians 5:23 underscores that God desires us to be whole in spirit, mind, and body.

Psalm 34:18: "The Lord is nigh unto them that are of a broken heart; and saveth such as be of a contrite spirit."

Matthew 11:28-30: "Come unto me, all ye that labour and are heavy laden, and I will give you rest. Take my yoke upon you, and learn of me; for I am meek and lowly in heart: and ye shall find rest unto your souls. For my yoke is easy, and my burden is light."

1 Peter 5:7: "Casting all your care upon him; for he careth for you."

2 Corinthians 1:3-4: "Blessed be God, even the Father of our Lord Jesus Christ, the Father of mercies, and the God of all comfort; Who comforteth us in all our tribulation, that we may be able to

comfort them which are in any trouble, by the comfort wherewith we ourselves are comforted of God."

While the Bible does not diagnose or provide modern treatment for mental health conditions, these verses demonstrate themes of comfort, understanding, and the importance of seeking support in times of emotional distress. Many faith-based communities and individuals use these passages as a foundation for discussions about mental health and the importance of seeking help when needed. Some faith communities have developed mental health ministries and programs to support individuals dealing with emotional and mental health challenges while incorporating these biblical principles. Interpretations of these passages may vary among individuals and religious denominations.

*"Casting all your care upon him;
for he careth for you."*

1 PETER 5:7

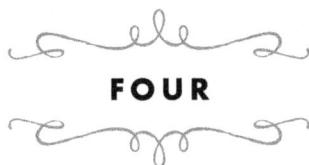

FOUR

Why Won't People Seek Help?

Numerous factors contribute to individuals avoiding seeking help, and as Christians, we must encourage them to prioritize their well-being. To achieve this, it is essential to understand why individuals often remain tight-lipped about their problems. While there are various reasons, we'll focus on a few key aspects.

Trust

Trust is a significant factor within our families, among friends, and concerning the openness of our problems. Many have experienced sharing confidential information with individuals they believed would keep their secrets, only to discover that these confidences were shared with others. The breach of trust is a common experience, making individuals hesitant to disclose their mental health issues. To address this, it is crucial to establish trust through clear communication. When considering sharing someone's struggles, seek permission and ensure the information will be handled with utmost confidentiality. Education and training within the church community can make it easier to help others while respecting their privacy.

Alienation

Feelings of alienation can deter individuals from sharing their concerns or illnesses. The fear of being left out or judged for mental health struggles often leads people to keep their issues to themselves. Creating an inclusive and supportive environment within the church is vital. Chapter One highlighted the impact of alienation on a young boy, emphasizing the need for awareness and empathy. By fostering a culture of acceptance and understanding, individuals may feel more comfortable seeking help without fearing being marginalized.

Grief

The global events of the past few years, especially the impact of COVID-19, have brought mental health to the forefront. Grief, stemming from various losses, has become a pervasive issue. The pandemic led to isolation, fear, and the loss of loved ones, creating a strain on individuals and families. Many have experienced profound grief, but the societal stigma around revealing this pain may prevent people from seeking help. Acknowledging the collective grief and normalizing discussions around mental health can encourage individuals to share their struggles without fear of judgment.

Fear of Job or Church Position Loss

The fear of repercussions regarding employment or church positions is another significant barrier to seeking help. Individuals may worry that admitting to mental health issues could lead to discrimination or exclusion. Within the church community, the desire to be accepted and maintain a favorable position can hinder openness about mental health struggles. It is essential to convey that the church is a safe space for everyone, regardless of their health status. Emphasizing acceptance and support can help break down these barriers and encourage individuals to prioritize their mental health.

Social Stigma

Social stigma remains a formidable obstacle to open discussions about mental health. Despite increasing awareness, misconceptions and unfavorable attitudes persist, leading individuals to conceal their struggles. The fear of being labeled, judged, or treated differently can hamper the willingness to seek help. As a church community, it is our responsibility to actively challenge and dismantle the stigma surrounding mental health. By fostering an environment that promotes understanding and empathy, we can create a space where individuals feel empowered to share their challenges without fear of discrimination.

Cultural Influences

Cultural factors also play a role in inhibiting help-seeking behaviors. Certain cultural norms may discourage individuals from discussing mental health openly. In some communities, mental health concerns are viewed as a personal failing rather than a medical condition. Churches must recognize and respect diverse cultural perspectives while actively working to change attitudes toward mental health. Education and awareness programs tailored to address cultural nuances can contribute to breaking down these barriers.

Lack of Awareness

Many individuals may avoid seeking help simply because they lack awareness of available resources or are unfamiliar with the signs and symptoms of mental health issues. The church can bridge this gap by providing education on mental health, conducting workshops, and disseminating information about available support services. A well-informed congregation is better equipped to recognize when someone may need help and can offer appropriate assistance.

Personal Denial

Individuals often grapple with their mental health challenges in silence due to personal denial. Admitting the need for help may be perceived as a weakness, leading some to suppress their struggles. The church can play a pivotal role in fostering an environment where vulnerability is embraced and seeking help is viewed as an act of strength. Personal testimonies and narratives shared within the church community can break down walls of denial and encourage others to seek the support they need.

In conclusion, the reluctance to seek help for mental health issues is a multifaceted challenge influenced by trust issues, feelings of alienation, grief, fear of repercussions, social stigma, cultural influences, lack of awareness, and personal denial. Addressing these factors as a church community requires a comprehensive approach involving education, destigmatization efforts, and creating an inclusive and supportive atmosphere. By actively engaging with these issues, the church can fulfill its role as a beacon of compassion, understanding, and encouragement, guiding individuals toward healing and wholeness.

"The Lord also will be a refuge for the oppressed, a refuge in times of trouble."

PSALMS 9:9

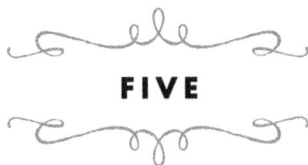

FIVE

The Path to Recovery: Seeking Help and Restoration

The question that often lingers in the minds of those silently grappling with mental health issues or substance use problems is whether they can truly get better if they seek help. The fear of never fully recovering or regaining a sense of normalcy often holds them back. It is a belief ingrained in many that they cannot escape the clutches of these conditions. But let me assure you, recovery is possible and a fundamental part of the healing journey.

What is Recovery?

Recovery from mental disorders and substance abuse disorders is a transformative process. It entails individuals actively working to improve their health and overall wellness, charting a self-directed path, and striving to realize their full potential. When we speak of recovery, we envision individuals reclaiming what they have lost—jobs, homes, families, and more.

In our role as trained volunteers, our mission goes beyond merely facilitating access to treatment. It extends to providing individuals with opportunities, a helping hand, and a place within the church community. Engaging them in church activities, such as participating in committees or contributing to the food pantry, can impart a sense of purpose. By involving individuals in these meaningful roles, we empower them and alleviate the feeling of invisibility that often accompanies their suffering.

Encouraging people to seek help is a crucial step in this process. We must convey to them that recovery is attainable despite the societal stigmas and fears that hinder disclosure. Many refrain from seeking help, fearing job loss, strained friendships, or the erosion of respect in the eyes of others. Our task is to assure them that recovery and a shared concern are possible. As we visit and comfort the afflicted, we must ensure that those facing mental health challenges feel embraced and integrated into the church community.

In addition to mental health issues, many individuals grapple with opioid addiction. To understand recovery fully, we must recognize addiction as a treatable condition. "Opioid Use Disorder (OUD) is a chronic and relapsing disease that affects countless lives."[2] Communities are grappling with its widespread impact. If you or someone you know is struggling with OUD, it is essential to acknowledge that treatment is available and recovery is within reach.

---

[2] www.yalemedicine.org

Supporting Recovery Through Inclusion and Responsibility

To help individuals struggling with behavioral health issues, it is crucial that we extend an inclusive and accepting hand within our community. People thrive when they feel included, embraced, and surrounded by individuals who care for them. Managing addictive behaviors can be daunting, but by involving them in church and community activities, we can offer them a sense of responsibility that can contribute to their overall well-being. This shared sense of purpose can help individuals regain control over their lives, counterbalancing the feelings of powerlessness often experienced during addiction.

Take my sister, for example, who battled drug addiction. Despite multiple treatment attempts, she would relapse upon returning to her everyday life. However, her relationship with the church became a lifeline. She secretly sent letters to the congregation, unbeknownst to her family, requesting their prayers and support. The church clerk read each request aloud, and she was welcomed with warmth and love when she attended church. Whenever she attended our church, they included her in events and group activities, and even when seen on the streets, she received warm embraces and genuine expressions of care. This unwavering, non-judgmental love saved her life. Even after a decade of sobriety, she remains actively engaged with the church, ready to contribute her cooking skills whenever needed. The memory of their compassionate support remains with her.

Being part of a church or community can be like a cool drink of water on a scorching day. It cools and comforts, offering a sense of belonging to individuals who may have felt disconnected from the world due to addiction or untreated mental health issues. Many individuals turn to the church when they struggle to connect with others, seeking the solace and support they believe can be found within its walls.

Individuals with behavioral health issues must be encouraged to actively participate in their recovery journey. They must be allowed to make decisions, take responsibility for their lives, and be a part of the healing process. While the road to recovery may be paved with challenges, the desire for improvement and change drives it. They may stumble and seek support repeatedly, but their relentless pursuit of health ultimately leads to recovery. It is crucial to remember that fear of failure is one of the most significant barriers individuals face when considering seeking help for behavioral health issues.

Recovery is about reclaiming what was lost—jobs, homes, families, or a sense of normalcy. Our role as trained volunteers extends beyond treatment facilitation; it is about offering support, opportunities, and a place within the church community. By extending our compassionate and accepting hand, we empower individuals to overcome challenges and regain control over their lives.

The church can play a pivotal role in this process, offering solace, a sense of belonging, and the unwavering love that many individuals desperately need. As we work together, embracing those in need, we can build a stronger, more inclusive, and compassionate community where recovery is possible and a reality.

"Is any sick among you? let him call for the elders of the church; and let them pray over him, anointing him with oil in the name of the Lord."

JAMES 5:14

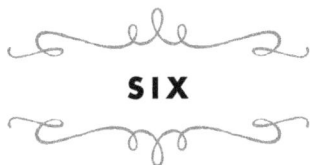

SIX

How to Build a Team for Your Mental Health Ministry

Establishing a team for your mental health ministry begins with the pastor. Setting the right tone and priorities is essential. From the pulpit, the conversation surrounding mental health should be elevated to a position of prominence. The congregation needs assurance that the church is committed to fostering a mental health component and the reasons behind it. Once this foundation is established, the pastor can move forward with selecting a team to represent the church in this vital department.

The pastor's understanding of the congregation's needs is paramount. In the event that they are still determining these needs, they should make a concerted effort to identify issues that congregants are concerned about while developing appropriate programs. The pastor must then introduce these plans to the church, explaining the reasons behind addressing these issues, which often affect families and the community. When individuals comprehend the purpose behind these initiatives, their interest in participating is piqued.

In the selection process for the team representing the church in this new endeavor, there are several characteristics the pastor should consider.

1. Confidentiality: A critical attribute necessary for building a program is confidentiality. People are often reluctant to share information when they fear their personal matters will be disclosed. Gossip can cause significant harm, leading to members leaving the church, losing trust, and withdrawing. Pastors must choose individuals with no reputation for gossiping about their fellow church members, as this could undermine the program's success.

2. Trust: Trust is vital in establishing meaningful relationships. It can either strengthen or weaken relationships. Given the stigma surrounding behavioral health issues and the reluctance of individuals to seek help, it is crucial not to include team members who may compromise the trust-building process by acting untruthfully or failing to seek forgiveness when they err. A trustful and empathetic relationship is the foundation of adequate support.

3. Interest in Learning: Successful programs require individuals who are eager to engage in ongoing educational opportunities. With substance use, opioid addiction, and mental health issues, knowledge is ever-evolving. The types of drugs change, methods of distribution shift, treatment approaches evolve, and, most importantly, people change. Staying up-to-date with current developments and participating in training are essential to maintaining an effective helping relationship.

4. Servant Attitude: Hebrews 13:16 emphasizes doing good and communicating, which pleases God. A servant's attitude signifies a willingness to help others, which aligns with God's desires. Aspiring to be a blessing to others and showing willingness to support those in need is essential. A servant's attitude allows God's work to manifest through our actions, ultimately helping individuals find healing and blessing in their lives.

5. Patience: Patience is a fundamental quality when assisting others. Significant behavioral changes do not occur overnight. Individuals need time to overcome challenges, which can be slow. It is important to exhibit patience when individuals do not change as quickly as one might hope. Patience is a valuable virtue, especially when it comes to behavioral health issues, as it takes time and effort to recover.

These characteristics form the foundation of individuals who can serve effectively in your mental health ministry. However, pastors and teams can always tailor the criteria based on the church's doctrines and principles. The key is to select individuals who genuinely want to help those in need.

A Personal Testimony: The Power of the Church in Recovery

Allow me to share a personal story that underscores the importance of the church in the recovery process. When my younger brother became ensnared by drug addiction during his teenage years, it was a series of life-altering events that led him down that path. In 1988, our parents' home caught fire, displacing them. While awaiting insurance resolutions, we invited them to live with my husband and me, a forty-five-minute drive from their city. Given the residency requirements, enrolling my brother in school in St. Louis, Missouri, proved challenging, as he was officially an East St. Louis, Illinois resident. We faced numerous legal hurdles, including securing legal custody and pursuing guardianship. It was a complex process, so my parents agreed that he would temporarily stay with a family friend, who was not a part of the street scene but rather a police officer raising his children. It was an environment we believed to be the right one for him.

However, the rise of crack cocaine affected both my brother and the police officer's daughter. When our parents returned home six months later, my brother was fundamentally changed. They had seen and talked to him often while he was away, but they were unprepared for their youngest child to be trapped in the clutches of addiction. Neither our family nor the police officer's family saw it coming. He was raised in a Christian environment and attended church regularly. Our parents had taught him right from wrong. Despite the seemingly ideal circumstances, he succumbed to drugs.

We tried everything we could to help him, but ultimately, his relationship with God and the church saved him. He grew tired of suffering, leaned on God, and asked for help. Our church services were on Saturdays since we are Adventists. However, my brother began attending different churches throughout the week, such as Baptist, Adventist, AME, CME, and Methodist, rotating through them. These churches offered him prayers and support. Friends and pastors from different denominations would inform me that my brother had worshipped with them. After a few months, he was cleansed by the grace of God and the supportive people in the churches who welcomed him with open arms. He also took the initiative to enroll in treatment to ensure he remained clean.

Conversations with individuals who have overcome addiction often reveal that the church and its members played a significant role in their recovery. This exemplifies the essence of being a faithful servant. In Acts 20:35, it is written, "I have shewed you all things, how that so labouring ye ought to support the weak, and to remember the words of the Lord Jesus, how he said, It is more blessed to give than to receive."

As Christians, we must support the weak and help them overcome their challenges, allowing them the opportunity to meet Jesus. Establishing a physical health department and a behavioral health ministry is essential to fulfilling this ministry and demonstrating God's love and compassion.

"Confess your faults one to another, and pray one for another, that ye may be healed."

JAMES 5:16

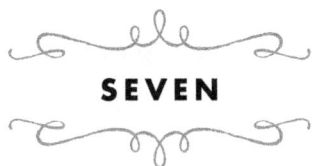

SEVEN

Setting up Your Partnership Leaders

Selecting the right team of Partnership Leaders is critical in establishing an effective support system for those in need. The team you assemble should comprise individuals the members can trust and respect. These individuals should be willing to connect with others and genuinely desire to spend time helping those in the community. In essence, they should possess the attitude of servants, ready and willing to provide assistance.

Your team of Partnership Leaders should be the go-to individuals within your faith-based community. They are dedicated workers who follow through with commitment and enthusiasm when entrusted with a task. These individuals are essential pillars in your program, and their qualities should include a solid commitment to the cause, the ability to work harmoniously with others, and leadership skills derived from their willingness to help.

Qualities of Effective Partnership Leaders

Commitment to the Cause: Your chosen leaders must have a profound commitment to the mission of your mental health ministry. This commitment goes beyond obligation; it reflects a deep desire to see people thrive and lead fulfilling lives.

Harmonious Teamwork: Effective Partnership Leaders should be capable of working harmoniously with others. Their ability to collaborate seamlessly within the team is crucial for the success of your program.

Leadership Skills: In this context, leadership stems from the willingness to help. Your leaders should inspire and guide others in the community toward positive change and support. They are the examples others can look up to.

Professional Backgrounds: Some leaders may have backgrounds in helping professions, such as behavioral health, counseling, or therapy. Their professional expertise can add valuable insight and skills to the team.

Continuous Learning: The field of behavioral health is ever-evolving. Leaders should demonstrate a willingness to keep their skills updated through ongoing learning. Regular training ensures they provide the most current and valuable services to those in need.

Identifying Potential Leaders

Consider the various departments within your church and identify individuals known as *go-getters* with specific specializations. Seek those who excel in offering support and care to those in need. However, it is essential to ensure that your team members align with the goals and values of your program, respecting established rules and guidelines. They should be committed to working as a team, possess strong organizational skills, and maintain positive interpersonal relationships.

The name "Partnership Team" signifies the essence of this group—people working together as partners to facilitate positive change. Their mission is to provide valuable services and information to assist others. They work collectively to enhance and improve the lives of those who seek their support.

Building a team of dedicated Partnership Leaders is an investment in the success of your mental health ministry. Their collective efforts will significantly create a supportive and transformative environment within your faith-based community.

"Be kindly affectioned one to another with brotherly love; in honour preferring one another."

ROMANS 12:10

EIGHT

Setting the Tone

Once the pastor decides on the characteristics he is looking for to participate in this ministry, he must ensure that he can have a good relationship with the people he selects. This means he does check-ins if he is not available to attend group meetings regularly. The pastor needs to know if the program is working, and the people in the group need to know that the church is supporting them—some questions to consider.

- What is the relationship between the group and the information being shared?
- Will the pastor want regular details?
- Would the pastor want to know the different needs of those seeking help?
- Does the pastor want names so he can pray for them?
- Do the members need to sign something with the people seeking help so that the team can share information and the

pastor can help ensure they have enough resources to help? This could be a confidentiality clause.

The pastor will need to work with the team on establishing ground rules. Ground rules are important in setting the tone and being organized. To develop a strong program, all involved must be on one accord.

What are the ground rules? Ground rules set the tone and expectations of the church and its leaders. It lets congregants know how to treat information, activities, and the members who seek help. For instance, confidentiality is important. When people are confiding to you, this information cannot be shared with others without the consent of the person sharing their information. Respect others and avoid behaviors that intimidate other members are some additional ground rules. Ground rules can be simple, such as requiring cell phones to vibrate during meetings or attend meetings on time. Once people know the rules, it gives them an opportunity to comply or leave the group.

Setting the tone ensures that all participants have a shared understanding of the purpose of their involvement and are aware of what is expected from them.

Some things to consider are the time issues.

- What time will meetings start?
- How long will the typical meeting last? (This is my suggestion. If you are going to have a start, there should be an expected end so attendees will have some idea how much time they need to allot for a meeting.)

- How often will you meet?

- How often are team members expected to host mental health activities (i.e., monthly, quarterly, or should there be a set number of yearly activities?

- What are the expectations of the members of the church? Assuming there are expectations.

- How often should the rules be updated?

- What reason(s) can committee members be removed?

- Will there be co-sponsored activities with local organizations?

- Is there a designated leader, or are we equally participating?

- Can information and activities be shared with those who do not attend your church?

This is the kind of information you should discuss before finalizing your team selection. It would be beneficial if they were informed of the committee's expectations. Knowing the team's goals, rules, and expectations will give people the opportunity to decide if they want to participate.

Team members and congregants should understand the goals of the new ministry so they can honor the rules and know what they are involved in. For instance, do you want to provide information on mental health to help families find resources? Do you want members to become more aware of behavioral health issues? Do you want to increase the number of people who will attend counseling? As a church, what is the end game? After the tone is set, how will the partnership team support the church's new behavioral health ministry?

"As every man hath received the gift, even so, minister the same one to another, as good stewards of the manifold grace of God."

1 PETER 4:10

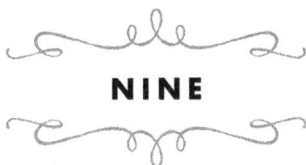

NINE

What Services Will the Team Provide?

Defining the services your team will provide is a fundamental step in your program, but extending beyond the basics is equally important. Consider the skills and expertise of your team members. Are they certified to counsel, licensed as therapists, or skilled in resource allocation? These services are pivotal to helping those in need. If your volunteers do not possess these skills, they must have the resources or knowledge to access them on behalf of others.

Diverse Backgrounds, Comprehensive Support

For instance, envision your team consisting of individuals with diverse backgrounds, such as a doctor and nurse practitioner with expertise in mental health, a social worker, and someone who retired from a career in mental health services. Each member contributes unique skills and knowledge to provide a comprehensive support system. This approach ensures a holistic and well-rounded approach to addressing behavioral health challenges within your community.

Valuable Contributions from Every Corner

It is important to recognize individuals who may not possess formal qualifications but have an innate ability to be team players and offer valuable support. These individuals might be quick learners, possess a servant's attitude, and are willing to learn from the team. Their life experiences and empathetic nature can make meaningful contributions to your program. By embracing diversity within your team, you enhance your ability to connect with and support a broad range of individuals within your community.

Training and Characteristics for Success

Remember that your Partnership Team provides direct services and is responsible for training others within the church community. When considering potential team members, look for characteristics like trustworthiness, a commitment to ongoing training, and a genuinely supportive attitude toward others. Additionally, understanding the effects of trauma is crucial for adequate support. Members should be empathetic and knowledgeable in this area.

Establishing Professional Boundaries

As your team engages in the sensitive work of behavioral health support, it is critical to establish and maintain professional boundaries.

While recognizing shared experiences, trauma bonding must not compromise the professional dynamic. Set clear boundaries to ensure a healthy and sustainable support system:

No Calls After Work: Avoid work-related calls or discussions after working hours to ensure a healthy work-life balance.

No Visiting at Their Home: Maintain professional boundaries by avoiding home visits and keeping interactions within appropriate settings.

Be Emotionally Prepared: Be prepared to handle emotionally charged situations and provide support without compromising your well-being.

Know Your Strengths: Recognize and use your strengths to benefit those you assist.

Know Your Weaknesses: Be aware of your limitations and seek assistance when needed.

Know Your Limitations: Understand when a situation requires professional intervention and your limitations in providing help.

By setting up a team of Partnership Leaders with these attributes and considerations in mind, you can establish a strong and effective support system within your faith-based community. Your team's dedication to learning, empathy, and maintaining professional boundaries will contribute to the overall success of your program, ensuring it meets the diverse needs of your community.

"But if ye have respect to persons, ye commit sin, and are convinced of the law as transgressors."

JAMES 2:9

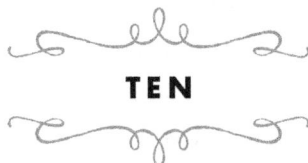

TEN

Do's and Don'ts as a Partnership Team Member

As a vital member of the Partnership Team, your role is instrumental in guiding and supporting individuals on their journey to deepen their relationship with God while fortifying their mental and emotional well-being. Maintaining a professional relationship with the individuals you assist is crucial to building trust and fostering a positive experience for both parties. Remember, your actions, whether positive or negative, have an impact, and they resonate within the community.

As you embark on this meaningful journey of aiding others, consider the profound significance of your work. Galatians 6:2 implores, "Bear ye one another's burdens, and so fulfill the law of Christ." Moreover, 2 Corinthians 1 reminds us that God comforts us so that we can, in turn, comfort others. Engaging in this work aligns with God's expectations of us, as we are made in His image. Therefore, loving one another is paramount, just as God loves us.

Do's

Respect Each Other: Respect forms the fundamental cornerstone of any relationship, including your role as a Partnership Team member. Always treat everyone with the utmost respect, particularly the person you are partnered with. Respect fosters trust and paves the way for a positive and productive partnership.

Represent Yourself Professionally: Your role as a Partnership Team member represents your faith and commitment to God. In all your interactions, conduct yourself with professionalism, integrity, and a solid commitment to your faith.

Demonstrate Your Commitment to God: Your dedication to God is the driving force behind your role. Ensure your actions reflect your unwavering commitment to your faith, serving as an example for those you assist.

Stick to Your Goals: Maintain a clear focus on your goals as a Partnership Team member. Whether your objectives involve aiding individuals in their spiritual journey or addressing mental health issues, staying goal-oriented is crucial to your effectiveness.

Don'ts

Don't Speak Negatively to the Person: Avoid speaking negatively to or about the person you are assisting. Negative words can have a detrimental impact on their mental and emotional well-being. Instead, provide encouragement and support to uplift their spirits.

Don't Share Their Personal Information with Others: Confidentiality is paramount in your role. Never share the personal information or experiences of the person you are assisting with anyone else unless you have their explicit consent.

Be Timely for Appointments: Respect the time and commitments of the person you assist by being punctual for your appointments. Being on time demonstrates your dedication to their well-being and helps build trust.

In summary, your role as a Partnership Team member is sacred, carrying great responsibility. Adhering to these do's and don'ts ensures that your efforts are guided by love, respect, and professionalism. Your commitment to God's work is a testament to your faith and a source of hope and support for those seeking your guidance and partnership. Ultimately, the positive impact you make reflects the love that God has for all of us.

"Wherefore comfort yourselves together, and edify one another, even as also ye do."

1 THESSALONIANS 5:11

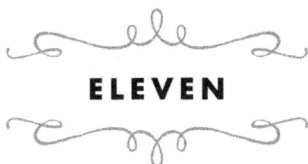

ELEVEN

Crafting a Sanctuary for Mental Wellness

Creating a safe and comforting space is crucial in your endeavor to champion mental wellness within your faith-based community. This sanctuary should be a haven for individuals in crisis, those seeking a moment of respite, or those requiring a confidential and secure place to gather their thoughts. Establishing such a space is paramount, as it cultivates an environment where people feel at ease to open up and seek support for their mental health challenges.

Let's delve into the key elements for crafting a haven within your church, ensuring that individuals feel welcomed and secure when sharing their experiences or seeking help.

Group 1: Designating the Physical Oasis

To initiate this journey, identify a specific area within your church premises that can serve as a safe space for meetings and support. This area should be easily accessible and ideally situated in a serene area of the church, away from the hustle and bustle of daily activities. Consider repurposing an existing room or establishing a new area, depending on the available resources.

Questions to ponder:

Where will this sanctuary be located in your church?

Pinpoint a suitable location that aligns with the church's layout and ensures privacy.

Group 2: Adorning Your Refuge

The subsequent step involves furnishing this space with items that promote comfort, relaxation, and functionality. Consider including a cozy chair, comfortable seating arrangements, a coffee pot, refreshments, tables for meetings and discussions, a small refrigerator stocked with water, and a bookshelf with relevant literature. Collectively, these elements contribute to transforming the space into a welcoming and supportive environment.

Questions to mull over:

What elements will you introduce to your safe space?

Outline the necessary items and furnishings to transform the space into a comforting and calming haven.

Group 3: Regulating Access and Informing the Congregation

To ensure that this safe space fulfills its intended purpose, careful consideration must be given to who will have access and how the congregation will be informed of its existence. Confidentiality and privacy are paramount in creating an environment where individuals can freely share their experiences.

Questions to address:

Who will have access to this sanctuary?

Define the individuals or groups allowed access and set clear guidelines.

How will you inform the congregation about the sanctuary?

Determine the best method for spreading the word about the safe space while respecting the need for discretion.

Group 4: Navigating Crisis Scenarios

A critical facet of your safe space is its capacity to provide immediate support in crisis situations. Envision a scenario where someone undergoes an anxiety attack during a church service. Knowing how to respond swiftly and effectively is imperative.

Questions for consideration:

Someone has an anxiety attack during service. How would you handle that?

Develop a protocol for dealing with mental health crises within the church, encompassing providing support, ensuring privacy, and seeking medical assistance, if necessary.

In summation, crafting a sanctuary for mental wellness within your church is a compassionate and significant step toward fostering a supportive environment for individuals grappling with mental health challenges. By addressing the physical space, furnishings, access management, and crisis-handling procedures, you can establish a space that encourages open conversations and provides a refuge for those in need. This safe space is pivotal in dismantling the stigma associated with mental health, fostering a sense of community, and nurturing understanding within your faith-based congregation.

"And let us consider one another to provoke unto love and to good works: Not forsaking the assembling of ourselves together, as the manner of some is; but exhorting one another: and so much the more, as ye see the day approaching."

HEBREWS 10:24-25

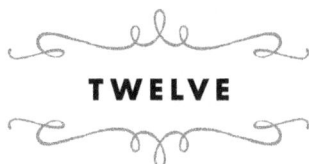

TWELVE

Developing a Comprehensive Church Safety Plan

C reating a comprehensive safety plan for your church goes beyond physical security; it encompasses protocols for handling medical and mental health crises. This chapter explores the significance of establishing a safety plan within your faith-based community and outlines vital components to ensure the well-being and security of your congregants.

1. Identifying the Safety Team

In the initial stages of developing a church safety plan, designate a safety team comprising individuals trained in emergency response, first aid, and mental health crisis intervention. Diversity within the team, including men and women, is crucial to effectively addressing various potential scenarios.

2. Introducing the Team to the Congregation

Introduce the safety team to the congregation, a task best undertaken by the pastor or church leadership. This introduction not only familiarizes the congregation with the team members but also instills a sense of reassurance and transparency regarding safety measures within the church.

3. Handling Medical Emergencies

Medical Crisis Response:

The safety team should follow a clearly defined protocol in a medical emergency. This protocol includes identifying the person responsible for responding to the crisis, devising a plan for removing the affected person from the sanctuary, and ensuring the availability of necessary equipment, such as wheelchairs.

Securing the Affected Individual:

Designate a secure and private location within the church for providing emergency assistance. Equip this space with essential medical supplies and equipment to ensure the affected individual receives prompt care.

4. Coordinating with Emergency Services

Contacting Emergency Services:

Train the safety team to promptly contact emergency services, whether it is an ambulance or the community mental health mobile unit, when a medical crisis occurs. Training and keeping the team informed of quick local resources ensures that professional help is coming as soon as possible.

Ensuring Safety During Crisis:

Maintaining a safe environment for all congregants may require security measures in certain situations. Having a team capable of providing physical support and assistance can be invaluable.

5. Boundaries and Non-Medical Intervention

The safety team should be well-versed in maintaining professional boundaries, especially when dealing with mental health crises. They should understand what actions they can and cannot take in terms of non-medical intervention. This involves ensuring the safety and well-being of the affected person while respecting their rights and dignity.

In summary, creating a church safety plan is essential to ensuring your congregants' well-being. A well-structured plan covering medical crises, including mental health emergencies, can provide a sense of security and support for the entire church community. By identifying the safety team, introducing them to the congregation, establishing clear protocols, and maintaining professional boundaries, your church can be better prepared to handle emergencies and crises effectively.

"Beloved, I wish above all things that thou mayest prosper and be in health, even as thy soul prospereth."

3 JOHN 1:2

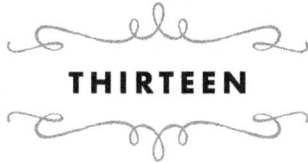

THIRTEEN

Plan of Action

After assembling your team, it is imperative to establish a comprehensive plan of action for your Behavioral Health Ministry. This plan will serve as a roadmap, guiding your team's efforts to break down behavioral health barriers within your faith-based community. Let's delve into the key components of your plan.

Setting Dates and Meeting Frequencies

Begin by scheduling dates for your team meetings. Determine how often these meetings will occur, whether weekly, bi-weekly, or monthly. Consistent and regular meetings foster cohesion and collaboration among team members.

Selecting Leadership Roles

Designate a leader and a secretary within your team. The leader will provide guidance and direction, while the secretary will maintain organized records, including contact information of individuals assisted. A designated leader ensures continuity if team members change or unforeseen circumstances occur.

Record Keeping for Accountability

While avoiding unnecessary paperwork, implement a system for recording key information. Recordkeeping could include tracking whom you've assisted, the nature of the help provided, and the outcomes. This recordkeeping ensures accountability and becomes valuable during team member transitions.

Problem-Solving Meetings

Schedule regular troubleshooting sessions. These meetings allow your team to address challenges, brainstorm solutions, and enhance the effectiveness of your ministry. Open communication is critical to overcoming obstacles and adapting to the evolving needs of those you serve.

Utilizing Existing Resources

Leverage the skills and expertise within your church community. If individuals have backgrounds in social work, substance use, or related fields, consider involving them to lighten the load and enhance the range of services your ministry can offer.

Confidentiality Measures

Whether utilizing paperwork or digital systems, maintain the highest level of confidentiality for individuals seeking assistance. If employing physical documents, secure them in a locked binder with limited access. Both the leader and secretary should uphold strict confidentiality standards.

Setting Goals for the Behavioral Health Ministry

As your ministry endeavors to eradicate mental health stigma, articulate clear and meaningful goals. The following are sample goals to guide your mission:

Goal 1: Promote Awareness and Education

Objective: Conduct regular educational sessions, workshops, and seminars within the church community to enhance understanding and diminish the stigma surrounding mental health issues.

Goal 2: Support and Counseling Services

Objective: Establish a safe and confidential space within the church for individuals to access counseling and support services for their mental health challenges.

Goal 3: Community Outreach and Advocacy

Objective: Actively engage with the broader community through outreach programs, events, and advocacy efforts to reduce mental health stigma and promote well-being.

By aligning your team with these goals, your Behavioral Health Ministry will navigate its mission with purpose, creating a compassionate and understanding environment within your faith-based community and beyond. These objectives will guide your actions and serve as a yardstick to measure your progress.

"Heal me, O LORD, and I shall be healed; save me, and I shall be saved: for thou art my praise."

JEREMIAH 17:14

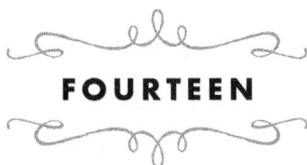

FOURTEEN

Getting Started

E mbarking on the journey of establishing a ministry to support your congregation is a significant decision that can bring about positive change within your faith community. Careful planning and effective communication are essential to ensure a successful start.

Pastoral Address

Begin by having the pastor address the congregation from the pulpit about the importance of mental health. Speaking from the pulpit provides a platform to highlight the significance of the upcoming ministry and sets the tone for open conversations within the church.

Announcement of the Plan

Make a clear and concise announcement from the pulpit outlining the plan for the new ministry. Share the vision, objectives, and the role the congregation can play. This announcement not only creates awareness but also invites participation.

Sign-Up Sheet

Encourage those with relevant experience or a passion for mental health to sign up on the church's bulletin board. Emphasize that while not everyone may be able to participate due to limited volunteer slots, the willingness to contribute is highly valued.

Volunteer Criteria

Communicate the criteria for volunteers. Express the need for individuals who are willing to volunteer their time and are eager to work with church members and community visitors. This criteria ensures a team with diverse skills and a shared commitment.

Orientation Importance

Stress the importance of the orientation process. Make it known that a professional will conduct the orientation, providing valuable insights into the ministry's goals and operations. Emphasize that the ministry is dedicated to listening, seeking resources, and creating a supportive environment but cannot provide diagnostic services.

Starting a ministry dedicated to mental health support is a transformative step for your congregation. By effectively communicating the plan, encouraging participation, and ensuring a thorough orientation, you set the stage for a ministry that can positively impact the well-being of your church community.

"Bear ye one another's burdens, and so fulfill the law of Christ."

GALATIANS 6:2

FIFTEEN

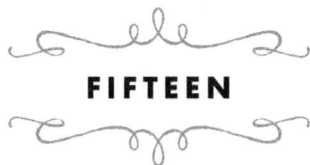

Pledging to Participate

Creating a pledge for all volunteers is a decisive step in solidifying your team's commitment to the mission of mental health support within your faith-based community. This pledge serves as a collective agreement, emphasizing the importance of unity, shared values, and responsible practices.

Here's a framework for developing and signing this meaningful pledge:

1. The Collective Pledge

Begin by crafting a collective pledge that encapsulates the core values and goals of your Mental Health Support Ministry. This pledge should reflect the shared commitment to breaking down barriers, fostering understanding, and providing compassionate support.

Example:

As Mental Health Support Ministry volunteers, we pledge to uphold the values of compassion, respect, and confidentiality. We commit to working collaboratively to create a safe and supportive space for individuals seeking mental health assistance.

2. Individual Commitments

The pledge encourages volunteers to include individual commitments or personal motivations for joining the ministry. The pledge adds a personal touch and reinforces the diverse strengths and perspectives within the team.

Example:

I pledge to bring empathy and understanding to every interaction, recognizing individuals' unique challenges. My commitment is to actively listen, learn, and contribute to the well-being of our church community.

3. Establishing Good Practices

Outline specific good practices that volunteers are expected to follow. These may include maintaining confidentiality, attending regular meetings, participating in ongoing training, and treating each individual with dignity and respect.

Example:

We pledge to maintain strict confidentiality regarding the personal information shared within the ministry. We commit to attending regular meetings, engaging in continuous learning, and treating everyone with dignity and respect.

4. Ceremony of Signing

Consider organizing a ceremony for the volunteers to sign the pledge physically. This activity could be a special moment during a church service or a dedicated event. The act of signing adds a symbolic weight to the commitment.

5. Displaying the Pledge

Once signed, prominently display the pledge within the ministry's designated space. Displaying the pledge serves as a visual reminder of the collective commitment and reinforces the importance of the mission.

6. Regular Review

Stress the importance of regularly reviewing and reaffirming the pledge as the ministry evolves. This ensures that the commitment to the mission remains strong and adapts to the community's changing needs.

By actively participating in the creation and endorsement of a significant pledge, volunteers showcase their unwavering commitment to the mission of the Mental Health Support Ministry. This unified dedication forms the bedrock of a united and influential team poised to bring about positive transformation in the lives of individuals

seeking support within your faith-based community. As you embark on this journey of commitment and establish various positive
programs, ensuring the inclusion of young people in your plans,
activities, and groups becomes crucial. Their integration enhances
the diversity of perspectives and ensures that your initiatives resonate
effectively with the diverse needs of the entire community. This
approach fosters a sense of belonging for the youth and enriches the
overall impact and relevance of the Mental Health Support Ministry.

"Chasten thy son while there is hope, and let not thy soul spare for his crying."

PROVERBS 19:18

SIXTEEN

Rising to the Challenge: Navigating the Mental Health Crisis Among Our Youth

In our nation, the crisis facing our youth has reached unprecedented levels, with crime rates soaring, leading to tragic outcomes such as arrests, fatalities, and incarcerations. Many parents desperately seek support and resources, only to discover that many communities lack the necessary services to assist them. The alarming increase in suicide rates among Black youth further compounds the urgency of addressing mental health challenges. Often overwhelmed and seeking refuge, parents turn to the one resource they know: the church. Churches must be a haven and well-equipped to provide the necessary assistance, making mental health preparation more vital than ever.

Historically, Black youth have faced barriers in accessing behavioral health (BH) treatment rooted in systemic inequities, social determinants of health, stigma, and mistrust of healthcare providers. A report from the Congressional Black Caucus in 2019 highlighted a crisis in Black youth suicide, revealing a near doubling of rates between 2007 and 2017 (Ring the Alarm, 2019).[3]

"The COVID-19 pandemic dealt a devastating blow to the mental well-being of youth, prompting the American Academy of Pediatrics to declare a "National State of Emergency in Children's Mental Health." This impact disproportionately affected communities of color, exacerbating stress, disruption, and grief. Black and Hispanic youth, in particular, faced a 2.5 times higher rate of losing a parent or caregiving adult to COVID-19 compared to their White counterparts." (Hidden Pain, Social Policy Analytics, 2021).[4]

"In St. Louis City, Black youth have weathered a "triple whammy" of high crime, the COVID pandemic, and racial tension over the past two years. According to local Black therapists, many youth have developed coping mechanisms that involve compartmentalizing emotions and disconnecting from the world around them (STL American, September 23, 2020)."[5] In such cases, Black youth may not even recognize the need for help or know how to seek it.

These grim statistics underscore the pressing need for churches to step up and address the mental health challenges faced by our youth. Through education, awareness, and proactive initiatives, churches can become pillars of support for a generation in crisis.

---

[3] Ring the Alarm, 2019

[4] Hidden Pain, Social Policy Analytics, 2021

[5] STL American, September 23, 2020

"Train up a child in the way he should go, and when he is old, he will not depart from it."

PROVERBS 22:6

Empowering Tomorrow: Nurturing Youth Leadership and Mental Well-being in the Church

The importance of addressing mental health issues among young people cannot be overstated, as they face an array of challenges that sometimes surpass those encountered by adults. Their limited understanding or coping capacities often make providing support and resources tailored to their needs even more crucial. The societal pressures on children and young adults are multifaceted, spanning issues like substance use within their families, struggles with drugs, anger, pain, grief, academic challenges, bullying, social isolation, financial and housing difficulties, and the absence of responsible parental figures. Additionally, some carry the burden of having drugs in their system from birth due to parents with addiction issues, compounding their challenges. Many also grapple with undiagnosed mental health concerns, experiencing feelings of profound sadness.

The church, ideally a place of refuge, sometimes faces barriers in reaching these young individuals, especially in an era dominated by social media where skepticism about organized religion prevails among some. Despite this, the imperative to extend help to these youth remains. Churches can play a pivotal role by implementing effective programs that attract and genuinely engage young people. Proverbs 22:6, although directed at parents, holds a broader truth – the need for collective efforts to guide the young generation in a positive direction. Churches should adopt a multifaceted approach to bridge the gap and effectively connect with young individuals. Opening the doors and inviting youth in is the first step, but inclusion in decision-making processes is equally crucial. Actively seeking their input on program and activity decisions ensures that the church remains relevant and responsive to their needs.

Here are some specific actions churches can take:

1. **Inclusion in Partnership Teams:** Young people should be integral members of the partnership teams, bringing their perspectives and insights to the table.
2. **Leadership Opportunities:** Empowering them to head up and plan activities allows them to take ownership and fosters a sense of responsibility.
3. **Active Leadership Roles:** Encouraging young individuals to take on leadership roles within the church promotes a sense of belonging and encourages personal and spiritual growth.
4. **Training Initiatives:** Training in mental health, conflict management, and leadership preparation equips them with valuable life skills. Regular training addresses

immediate concerns and contributes to their overall personal development.

5. By actively involving and investing in the younger generation, churches can create a nurturing environment that addresses mental health challenges and helps young individuals grow into responsible, resilient, and spiritually grounded adults.

"Lo, children are an heritage of the LORD: and the fruit of the womb is his reward."

PSALMS 127:3

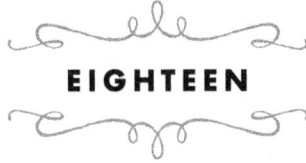

EIGHTEEN

Nurturing Mental Wellness in Youth

I n supporting teens facing mental health challenges, adults, churches, and family members play pivotal roles in fostering positive well-being. Here are additional strategies to empower young individuals on their journey to mental health:

- Empower Them to Create Their Wellness Plan:

Encourage teens to actively participate in developing their self-care and wellness plans. By taking ownership of their mental health strategies, they can personalize approaches that resonate with their needs and preferences. This sense of control can be empowering and promote a proactive approach to well-being.

- Challenge Stigmas and Promote Self-Care:

Instill the belief that self-care is fundamental to well-being. Empower teens to challenge societal stigmas surrounding mental health and advocate for their own mental well-being. By fostering a culture that normalizes self-care practices, young people can develop resilience and coping mechanisms to navigate life's challenges.

- Cultivate Positive Social Connections:

In a digital age where online friendships prevail, guiding teens in building meaningful, face-to-face connections is crucial. Encourage participation in church events and community gatherings, or introduce them to peers within your social circle. Establishing reliable support systems can help teens feel a sense of belonging and connectedness.

- Prioritize Mental Health Education:

Equip teens with knowledge about mental health, emphasizing the importance of destigmatizing conversations around it. Teach them coping skills such as breathing techniques and journaling to manage stress and express their emotions. Highlight the significance of seeking support from trusted adults or professionals when needed.

- Promote Healthy Lifestyle Practices:

Educate young people on the correlation between physical and mental well-being. Encourage activities that involve movement, outdoor exposure, regular exercise, and sufficient sleep. Collaborate with them to identify enjoyable and health-promoting activities that contribute to positive overall well-being.

- Facilitate Positive Relationships:

Foster partnerships with individuals who share similar goals and aspirations. Encourage collaborative efforts, emphasizing the importance of working together toward common objectives. Engaging with like-minded peers provides a sense of purpose and facilitates positive relationships.

By incorporating these strategies, adults and communities can actively contribute to creating an environment where teens feel supported, valued, and equipped with the tools to nurture their mental wellness.

FINAL SUMMARY

In today's dynamic world, challenging and transforming prevailing stigmas surrounding mental health, particularly within faith-based communities, is a critical endeavor. "Breaking Behavioral Health Barriers in Faith-based Communities" stands as a beacon of hope, providing a comprehensive guide to navigating these communities' complex mental health landscape. The journey begins in *Chapter One*, where the book addresses the historical negativity surrounding mental health, emphasizing the importance of understanding and acceptance in dispelling stereotypes and fostering healthier attitudes toward mental well-being.

The book underscores the urgent need for mental health awareness within faith communities. By delving into common disorders and symptoms, it empowers readers to recognize signs of mental health issues, calling individuals to action with a message of receptivity and compassion towards those grappling with such challenges. It goes further, challenging the prevailing silence around mental health, uncovering the reasons behind the secrecy, and highlighting the detrimental effects of such silence. The book advocates for open conversations as a powerful tool to cultivate understanding and acceptance.

"Breaking Behavioral Health Barriers in Faith-based Communities" effectively bridges the gap between faith and mental health, harmoniously promoting the coexistence of these two aspects. It emphasizes that seeking mental health support alongside spiritual guidance is not a betrayal of faith but a responsible approach to holistic well-being. The focus on faith-based ministries is a reminder that pastors, ministry leaders, and congregations must collaborate to create an environment where mental health is given the attention and care it deserves.

Building a supportive community takes center stage in the book, with inclusivity, open dialogue, and empathy highlighted as paramount. Readers are challenged to take tangible actions to create a caring environment within their faith communities. The guide provides practical insights on establishing a behavioral health ministry within a church, offering a roadmap enriched with valuable resources. It assists readers in setting faith-based goals for their ministry, ensuring a practical approach to supporting mental health within faith communities.

"Breaking Behavioral Health Barriers in Faith-based Communities" emerges as a timely and invaluable resource, calling on faith communities to prioritize the holistic well-being of their members, including their mental health. It transcends being a mere guide; it is a compelling call to action, empowering individuals and faith-based institutions to overcome stigma and cultivate a more inclusive and supportive environment for everyone who enters their doors.

A PERSONAL NOTE FROM THE AUTHOR

In the tapestry of life, it is awe-inspiring to reflect on how each thread, each moment, has been carefully woven by the divine hands of God. From my earliest memories of standing in the corner listening to my parents argue, to the pivotal moment of calling my uncle to intervene, every step seems purposeful. Little did I know that such experiences would shape my understanding of communication and conflict de-escalation.

God's guidance has been evident throughout my life, leading me to help countless individuals facing mental health challenges. For years, I navigated this field instinctively, unknowingly supporting those in crisis. From diffusing conflicts on and off the job to offering comfort in moments of despair, my journey has been marked by instances where mental health intersected with my path.

One particular incident during my college years remains etched in my memory. A fellow student, overwhelmed by the stark disparities between her family's narratives and the realities of college life, contemplated jumping from the top of our towering dorm building. In that critical moment, as if guided by divine intervention, I became a vessel of comfort, preventing a tragedy with words of solace and empathy.

Through the years, I've encountered individuals grappling with mental health issues, often hidden behind a facade of anger or distress. In one such instance, I intervened with an enraged employee on the verge of causing harm. Through conversation and understanding, I discovered the deep-rooted pain stemming from domestic violence that had haunted him since his youth. These encounters, guided by an inner compass, revealed my affinity for helping those facing mental health struggles.

My mother's teachings on mental health provided a solid foundation, and as I progressed in my career, I found myself drawn to this field. Stopping crises, offering support, and navigating the complexities of mental health became a calling that resonated deeply with me.

The prevalence of mental health stigma in my community, especially during the COVID-19 pandemic, propelled me to advocate for change. I spoke to thousands of congregants about establishing behavioral health ministries, sharing insights from my experiences. In 2015, I collaborated with The Behavioral Health Network of Greater St. Louis to co-create a model for reducing mental health stigma in faith-based communities. The success of the Bridges to Care & Recovery Program, which trained 114 congregations in St. Louis, Missouri, led to the adoption of the model in San Antonio, Texas.

Retiring as the Director of Faith-based Initiatives on December 31, 2022, was intended for cherished moments with family, especially my grandson. However, churches' persistent need for mental health education beckoned me back. The calling from pastors in my hometown in Illinois to resume training churches underscored the urgency for churches to be at the forefront of mental health ministry.

As communities turn to churches for various services, it is imperative for pastors and congregations to embrace the responsibility of mental health education. Beyond the traditional roles, churches can become beacons of support, offering resources and information to nurture the mental well-being of their members.

The journey continues, driven by a deep conviction that addressing mental health stigma in faith-based communities is not just a mission but a divine calling—one that echoes the profound love God has shown us and the transformative power we can collectively wield.

SAMPLE MENTAL HEALTH ACTIVITIES FOR CHURCHES

Rose Jackson-Beavers

1. Preach on mental health-related topics.
2. Display mental health materials in the vestibule.
3. Have a play on seeking support/a role play on helping someone.
4. Introduce local resources to church members.
5. Add a mental health message to your church bulletin.
6. Put something about mental health on your website.
7. During the month of May, have church members dress in green for Mental Health Awareness. Discuss green as being the mental health color.
8. Have a guest speaker talk about depression, anxiety, or mental illness.
9. Have a support group to deal with grief or depression.
10. Have a Zoom panel discussion with speakers.
11. Have a mental health brunch with a speaker.
12. Offer biblically-sound mental health education.
13. Open a mental health resource center.

14. Establish a suicide protection policy or other policies. Have your trained team work on them and share them with the church.

15. Use brain teaser games to introduce mental health symptoms or terminology. This can help people understand mental health.

16. Offer a training session on making calls to a hotline.

17. Have your members create a de-stress mental health room.

18. Create an activity like a Bible search for verses that support anxiety, stress, happiness, sadness, etc.

19. Invite your community to a mental health workshop.

20. Ask your members who have social media platforms if they would post mental health graphics on their Facebook pages, like hotline numbers.

21. Create a wellness newsletter and distribute it to your members with important phone numbers.

SUGGESTED CHURCH MENTAL HEALTH TRAINING TOPICS

- Breaking Behavioral Health Barriers in Faith-Based Community

- Signs and Symptoms of Mental Health

- Reducing the Stigma of Mental Health in Faith-based Communities

- Understanding and Creating Essential Partnerships

- Faith and Mental Health

- Communications and Interviewing Skills

- Mental Health and Substance Use

There are many topics that would be helpful in training churches to reduce the stigma of mental health. These topics are the ones that I train churches and their congregations on to give them the basic information to help others.

NATIONAL RESOURCES

- 988 Suicide & Crisis Lifeline

Depression Related Organizations/Sites

- National Suicide Prevention Lifeline – Only federally funded national hotline. Provides a 24-hour, toll-free, confidential crisis hotline for anyone (you or a loved one) who may be suicidal or in psychological crisis. Calls are routed to the nearest available crisis center in your area. Get immediate suicide crisis support, mental health information and referrals to services in your area.

Suicide/Crisis Hotline: (800) 273-TALK (8255)
Hotline for Spanish Speakers: (888) 628-9454
TTY Hotline: (800) 799-4TTY (4889)

- National Hope line Network – Provides a national, 24-hour, toll-free suicide prevention hotline. Your call will be connected to the nearest certified crisis center. You can also search for a crisis center nearest you in their online directory.

Suicide Hotline: (800)-SUICIDE (784-2433)
Kristin Brooks Hope Center
615 7th Street NE

Washington, DC 20002

Phone: 202.536.3200

Email (General Comments):

info@hopeline.com

• National Institute of Mental Health (NIMH) – Federal agency that provides mental health information, supports, and conducts research on mental and behavioral disorders.

National Institute of Mental Health (NIMH)

Public Information and Communications Branch

6001 Executive Boulevard, Room 8184, MSC 9663

Bethesda, MD 20892-9663

Main Local: (301) 443-4513

Main Toll-Free: (866) 615-6464

TTY Local: (301) 443-8431

TTY Toll-Free: (866) 415-8051

Fax: (301) 443-4279

Email: nimhinfo@nih.gov

• National Alliance on Mental Illness (NAMI) – Largest national grassroots organization dedicated to improving the lives of people with mental illness and their families. Provides support, education, advocacy, and research for people living with mental illness. Local chapters in every state.

2107 Wilson Blvd., Suite 300

Arlington, VA 22201-3042

Phone: (703) 524-7600

TDD: (703)-516-7227

Fax: (703) 524-9094

Help Line: 800-950-NAMI (6264)
Email: info@nami.org

- Mental Health American (formerly known as National Mental Health Association) – One of the nation's leading non-profit organizations committed to helping all people have better mental health. Provides advocacy and information on mental health disorders, treatment, tests and screenings and where to get help.

Mental Health America
2000 N. Beauregard Street, 6th Floor
Alexandria, Virginia 22311
Main: (703) 684-7722
Main Toll-Free: (800) 969-6MHA (6642)
TTY: (800) 433-5959
Fax: (703) 684-5968
Crisis Line: (800) 273-TALK (8255)
Email: Form on site

- Depression and Bipolar Support Alliance (DBSA) – Nation's leading non-profit organization supporting individuals with depression and bipolar disorder. DBSA has an 800 information and referral line, over 1,000 support groups nationwide, educational materials and programs. DBSA also supports research and promotes advocacy for people living with mood disorders.

Depression and Bipolar Support Alliance
730 N. Franklin Street, Suite 501
Chicago, Illinois 60610-7224
Toll-free: (800) 826-3632

Fax: (312) 642-7243
Email: info@dbsalliance.org

• American Foundation for Suicide Prevention – National organization, focused on the prevention of suicide. Provides education and research grants, programs for individuals surviving loss from suicide and advocacy for legislation to further research and suicide prevention. Has local chapters across the country.

• American Foundation for Suicide Prevention

120 Wall Street, 22nd Floor
New York, NY 10005
Toll-free: (888) 333-AFSP
Phone: (212) 363-3500
Fax: (212) 363-6237
Email: inquiry@afsp.org

• American Association of Suicidology (AAS) – Founded in 1968, a not-for-profit organization dedicated to the understanding and prevention of suicide. AAS promotes research, provides publications, public education, and awareness, training to professionals and support groups for survivors. AAS is a national clearinghouse for information on suicide.

American Association of Suicidology
5221 Wisconsin Avenue, NW
Washington, DC 20015
Phone: (202) 237-2280
Fax: (202) 237-2282
Email: info@suicidology.org

OTHER BOOKS BY ROSE

Journey to Jesus With Me
(30-Day Devotional with activities)

Each day is considered a gift, so treat yourself to the best gift of all: a stronger, more capable, and spiritual self.

"Journey to Jesus With Me" is a daily devotional by Rose Jackson-Beavers to 1) encourage you to look inwardly, 2) think about the things that might have been embedded in your subconscious, and 3) motivate you to make changes in your present.

For 30 days, this book guides the readers with a prominent daily scripture, allowing each person to address past thoughts with current actions. You will not go on this journey alone as Rose Jackson-Beavers relives some of her moments. Through transparency and faith, Rose shares lessons her mother instilled in her and how she incorporated those lessons into her life. She shares a corresponding scripture to help those who desire encouragement and help them think of those things.

This book was written to build the reader up and give you a fresh start to each day, no matter how the previous day has been. Within

30 days, allow yourself the space and opportunity to put your spiritual and emotional life first. Aim to fix the things that might be hindering you. As you go through each day with Rose, allow the scriptures, anecdotes, and thought-led questions to speak to you as you pursue life's trials. As each day passes, you get stronger until finally, you have your own stories to reference and build yourself up.

Bottled Up Inside:
African American Teens and Depression:

This book was co-written with Rev. Jermine Alberty.

Today's youth face numerous obstacles. It is incredible how they can keep so much bottled up. The pressures of today can often be so troubling that they are shaken to their core and may find themselves bursting at the seams from all the stuff they keep inside.

"Bottled Up Inside: African American Teens and Depression" seeks to educate and inform individuals who work with youth through the author's personal and professional lived experiences.

Depression is a huge health concern for African Americans due to a variety of issues affecting their families and communities. Too many people are not seeking help and treatment, and this has prevented many from healing due to the stigma associated with mental illness.

The suicide rate among Black teens is increasing, with this being the third leading cause of death for young people 15-24. It is essential to discuss the issues of mental health and how it affects people so when help is needed, people will not be afraid to ask for help.

In this book, the reader will learn how to assist youth dealing with the turmoil of adolescence, gain an understanding of depression, identify potential risk factors and protective factors, and learn an intervention to help youth in non-crisis and crisis situations.

ABOUT THE AUTHOR

Rose Jackson-Beavers is the author of 15 books. She advocates for teens and collaborates closely with others to encourage young people never to give up. She resides in Florissant, Missouri, with her family.

www.ingramcontent.com/pod-product-compliance
Lightning Source LLC
Chambersburg PA
CBHW030023290326
41934CB00005B/456